The
Nursing Mother's Companion
Breastfeeding
DIARY

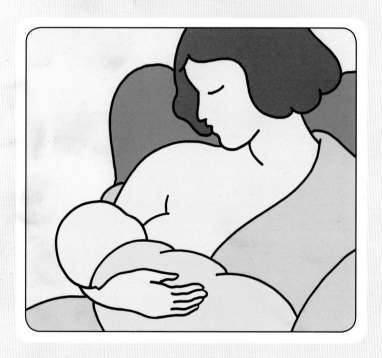

Kathleen Huggins
AND
Jan Ellen Brown

THE HARVARD COMMON PRESS
BOSTON, MASSACHUSETTS

The Harvard Common Press
535 Albany Street
Boston, Massachusetts 02118
www.harvardcommonpress.com

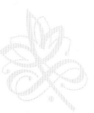

Printed in China
Printed on acid-free paper

Library of Congress Cataloging-in-Publication Data

Huggins, Kathleen.
    The nursing mother's companion breastfeeding diary / Kathleen
Huggins and Jan Ellen Brown.
        p. cm.
    ISBN 978-1-55832-730-6 (hc : alk. paper)
1. Breastfeeding--Popular works. 2. Mothers--Diaries. I. Brown,
    Jan Ellen. II. Title.
    RJ216.H845 2010 Suppl.
    649'.33—dc22

                                        2010005984

Special bulk-order discounts are available on this and other Harvard
Common Press books. Companies and organizations may purchase
books for premiums or resale, or may arrange a custom edition, by
contacting the Marketing Director at the address above.

Cover design by Suzanne Heiser
Text design by Deborah Kerner

10 9 8 7 6 5 4 3 2 1

Preface

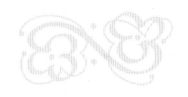

Congratulations on the birth of your baby!

We offer this diary to help you keep track of the first few months with your nursling, and, more important, to provide daily coaching for you as your baby grows. We hope the diary will also serve as a place to record your thoughts and observations, and later as a keepsake of the precious first weeks with your newborn.

Since I first wrote *The Nursing Mother's Companion*, more than twenty-five years ago, I have marveled at the many ways mothers find to keep track of their babies' feedings, diapers, and developmental progress. Breastfeeding is not science; the beauty of nursing is that it is instinctive and natural. Babies should be nursed without rules, according to their own cues. Yet almost all new mothers who come to see us bring along some kind of log. Whether it is on scrap paper, in a notebook, or on a homemade grid, a daily log of feedings and diaper changes gives many mothers confidence. In addition, as the American Academy of Pediatrics points out in its position paper on breastfeeding, a mother's log may help the doctor or lactation specialist identify problems that may arise with the baby.

So it made sense to create a nursing log book, both to help new mothers record daily feedings and diaper changes and to do one thing more: to provide day-by-day breastfeeding tips to usher mothers along. After all, the first few months set the stage for your nursing experience. Along with *The Nursing Mother's Companion*, the timely coaching here will help you get off to the best start.

As you make your way through this book, don't just record data; write down your thoughts and impressions, too. Someday this diary will be a precious reminder of your first days together with your baby.

—KATHLEEN HUGGINS

How to Use This Diary

tart the diary on the day your baby is born, at the page headed "Birth Day." If that day has already passed, start on whichever page corresponds with your baby's age. This way the daily breastfeeding tips will follow your baby's development.

For each day, you'll find a grid for tracking input (feedings) and output (wet and dirty diapers). The grid has space for twelve feedings per day; if you find you're nursing more frequently than this, record only the feedings that are more than just snacks. The first column is for noting the time that the feeding started; the second is for indicating which breast you started on (**L** or **R**), so you'll know to start the following feeding on the other side. In the columns headed **L** and **R**, you can estimate the time the baby spent actively nursing—that is, sucking and swallowing—on each side (you may prefer to skip this detail). If you elect or need to express milk, record the amount you collect under "Amount Expressed." If you give the baby a full or partial feeding of formula or pumped breast milk, you can note the amount you feed in either the column headed "Breast Milk" or the one headed "Formula." Finally, in the bottom row, marked "Totals," you can total your daily amounts. This will be particularly helpful if you are pumping or feeding expressed milk or formula.

Sample Grid

DAY AND DATE: *Tuesday April 12*

	TIME	START (L or R)	MINUTES L	R	AMOUNT EXPRESSED	SUPPLEMENT AMOUNT BREAST MILK	FORMULA	OUTPUT WET	POOP
1	*9 am*	*R*	*10 min*	*25 min*	*1 oz*			*x*	*x*
2									

The feeding started at 9:00 in the morning, on the right breast. After 25 minutes on the right, the baby nursed for 10 minutes on the left. Because the mother was slightly engorged, she expressed one ounce of milk to freeze for later use. She also changed a wet and dirty diaper. She will continue to record feedings on the same page until about the same time the next morning.

Opposite each grid is a page with an inspirational quote and some blank space. In the blank space you can note the baby's milestones, jot down your feelings about motherhood, write letters to your baby, list questions or concerns to share with the doctor, or record guests, gifts, cards, or phone calls you have received. Use this space as you like to create your own history of your and your baby's early weeks together.

DAY AND DATE: . . . .

		START	MINUTES		AMOUNT	SUPPLEMENT AMOUNT		OUTPUT	
	TIME	(L or R)	L	R	EXPRESSED	BREAST MILK	FORMULA	WET	POOP
1									
2									
3									
4									
5									
6									
7									
8									
9									
10									
11									
12									
	TOTALS:								

Birth Day. Happy Birthday! Congratulations on becoming a new mother. This diary will help guide you day by day as you navigate your baby's early days of breastfeeding.

Ask for a lot of help as you get started. Keep your baby close, skin to skin, and nurse often. Rest with the baby as much as you can.

Colostrum, your early milk, is your baby's first vaccine. Full of protein and antibodies, it will protect your baby from harmful bacteria and viruses.

A newborn baby has only three demands. They are warmth in the arms of its mother, food from her breasts, and security in the knowledge of her presence. Breastfeeding satisfies all three.

—*Grantly Dick-Read*

_____

_____

_____

_____

_____

_____

_____

_____

_____

_____

_____

_____

_____

_____

_____

_____

_____

_____

DAY AND DATE: ....

	TIME	START (L or R)	MINUTES		AMOUNT EXPRESSED	SUPPLEMENT AMOUNT		OUTPUT	
			L	R		BREAST MILK	FORMULA	WET	POOP
1									
2									
3									
4									
5									
6									
7									
8									
9									
10									
11									
12									
TOTALS:									

One Day Old. Is the fact that your baby is here starting to sink in?

Baby's early bowel movements are called meconium. These sticky, black early stools are passed as the baby ingests colostrum in the first few days.

When your baby awakes after a sleepy period, he may root about for your breast. Hold him against your bare skin so he will latch on to the breast more readily. Ask a nurse or lactation specialist to help you whenever you need assistance. Since you may be leaving the hospital soon, have your partner present during the lessons so he'll be able to help you at home.

If your baby is having difficulty latching on to the breast, if he was born three weeks or more early, or if you have had breast surgery in the past, have a staff member show you how to hand-express or pump your milk until it is clear that your milk supply is adequate and your baby is able to complete a feeding. Early, consistent breast stimulation and milk removal is the key to building your milk supply.

A little child born yesterday
A thing on mother's milk and kisses fed.

——Homer

_____

_____

_____

_____

_____

_____

_____

_____

_____

_____

_____

_____

_____

_____

_____

_____

_____

DAY and DATE: ....

	TIME	START (L or R)	MINUTES L	MINUTES R	AMOUNT EXPRESSED	SUPPLEMENT AMOUNT BREAST MILK	SUPPLEMENT AMOUNT FORMULA	OUTPUT WET	OUTPUT POOP
1									
2									
3									
4									
5									
6									
7									
8									
9									
10									
11									
12									
TOTALS:									

Two Days Old. Having a newborn may feel wonderful, but if the birth didn't happen as planned you may also feel disappointment and even anger. Resolve your feelings by talking about the delivery with your doctor, your partner, a friend, or a loving relative. Then move on and focus on your beautiful baby.

Don't be surprised if there are periods when your baby wants to nurse more frequently than usual. We call this cluster feeding. Cluster feeding often occurs in the night, and typically in the first night home from the hospital. Babies nurse quite often when they are thirsty or hungry or just need to suck. This behavior does not mean your baby "isn't getting enough."

It was the tiniest thing I ever decided to put
my whole life into.

—*Terri Guillemets*

_____

_____

_____

_____

_____

_____

_____

_____

_____

_____

_____

_____

_____

_____

_____

_____

_____

_____

_____

9a-9p day 3

DAY AND DATE: Sat. 12/24

	TIME	START (L or R)	MINUTES L	MINUTES R	AMOUNT EXPRESSED	SUPPLEMENT AMOUNT BREAST MILK	SUPPLEMENT AMOUNT FORMULA	OUTPUT WET	OUTPUT POOP
1									
2									
3									
4									
5									
6									
7									
8									
9									
10									
11									
12									
	TOTALS:								

Three Days Old. This day is full of changes.

You may be home or still in the hospital, but either way you are probably feeling the effects of the delivery—aching muscles, a tender perineum, or perhaps the discomfort of a cesarean incision—as well as tiredness from lack of sleep and mounting hormonal changes. Nap when you can, and try to limit visitors who could sap your time and energy. Your partner can be the gatekeeper. Stay in your PJs all day long, so that guests won't stay as long or expect as much.

Your breasts may be full and tight as they begin producing mature milk. This swelling is normal. You will want to keep the baby close and nurse as often as possible. Frequent feedings and cold packs after feedings will also help. If your baby has her "days and nights mixed up," she may tend to sleep long stretches during the day. In this case, wake her for feedings at two-and-a-half-hour intervals. This will limit your engorgement as well as help establish your milk supply.

Also on this day, the baby's stools will begin looking less tarry and more greenish-brown in color. She should have at least three wet diapers and three dirty ones today.

Mother love is the fuel that enables a normal human being
to do the impossible.

—*Marion C. Garretty*

Weignt 5.14 @ 1pm

3am pee
8:00 feed
10:15 "
12:00 feed
1:30 feed

10:30 large poop /pee
1:30 am pee ———▷

5-7min letdown
massaging — in beg.
10min

DAY AND DATE: ....

	TIME	START (L or R)	MINUTES L	MINUTES R	AMOUNT EXPRESSED	SUPPLEMENT AMOUNT BREAST MILK	SUPPLEMENT AMOUNT FORMULA	OUTPUT WET	OUTPUT POOP
1									
2									
3									
4									
5									
6									
7									
8									
9									
10									
11									
12									
	TOTALS:								

Four Days Old.

Few mothers anticipate the emotions that typically follow childbirth. Weepiness is common and normal. Other women may not tell you this, but "baby blues," generally experienced as an all-day crying jag, come to most new mothers on the fourth day post partum. Though you may think you should feel sheer bliss over the birth of your baby, adjusting to new motherhood isn't automatic or easy, and most women take at least several weeks to recover physically and emotionally and become comfortable in the care and feeding of their newborns.

Your partner is an important part of your nursing relationship. He can feed and comfort you as well as care for your newborn. Although he may not change a diaper as well as you, he is learning, and he will become more proficient with patience and practice.

Expect four wet diapers and four dirty ones in this 24-hour period.

weight 6.0 @ 11:15   102 3/4   4w 3cc
                                5-4 3 1/2 cc
1-1.5° apart   2-3 feedings   BREASTFEEDING DIARY   15
   cluster feed 7-8 AM close 11-12-1 3.5 oz
                          feed nap -12° P

The most important thing a father can do for his children
is to love their mother.

2:45 express 5ml   5/6 -8/9
4:30 express 7.5ml   —Theodore Hesburgh
9:00 "   7.5ml   2-3°
    →9:30 feed   feed @ mid
11:15 poop   1057 poop/pee?
11:35 express 5ml   1055 feed   poop
11:55   "   5ml   1230 feed   =96
12:15 feed   1230 express 10ml
12:30 pee/poop   230 poop/pee
1:15 express 5ml   245 feed
1:50   "   5ml   370 pump 10cc
2:00 feed x 5min (+4ml) 5:15 poop
2:28 express 4ml   5:35 feed
2:45   "   4ml   6:00 pump 5cc
4:15   "   7.5ml   7:40 poop/pee
4:25 feed   7:45 feed
4:30 pee/poop   8:15 expressed 10ml
5:50 express 12.5ml
6:25 feed
7:10 pee/poop (pump)
07:50 express 7.5ml   4 poops
8:30 poop/pee?   6 pees
8:35 feed
9:15 pumped 5ml
10:10 express

DAY and DATE:

	TIME	START (L or R)	MINUTES		AMOUNT EXPRESSED	SUPPLEMENT AMOUNT		OUTPUT	
			L	R		BREAST MILK	FORMULA	WET	POOP
1									
2									
3									
4									
5									
6									
7									
8									
9									
10									
11									
12									
	TOTALS:								

Five Days Old. Today you're likely to experience the peak of breast fullness as your milk "comes in." When you're nursing you should be able to hear the baby swallow, and your breasts should feel softer and lighter afterward. Let the baby completely soften one breast before switching to the other.

If your nipples are sore, find help in getting the baby latched on better. Get immediate help if your baby can't latch on at all or doesn't seem to suck effectively, in which case you may need to express your milk to build and maintain your supply. Feed your baby any expressed milk after nursing.

By Day Five, a baby's bowel movements are normally yellow, curdled- or seedy-looking, and loose. This is not diarrhea; loose yellow stools usually indicate that a baby is getting enough milk.

Your baby may have his first doctor's checkup today. Take this diary with you so you can report feeding intervals, diaper counts, and questions and concerns.

15ml x 8 = 120   poop / pee
                  |||| / |||| ||

Before you were conceived I wanted you.
Before you were born I loved you.
Before you were here an hour I would die for you.   total 123cc
This is the miracle of life.

—*Maureen Hawkins*

9:20 fed (R)   12:50 fed (L) x 15m
9:55 expressed 14ml   1:20 pump 10cc
11:20 poop/pee   1:45 fed (R) x 10m
11:30 fed (R)   2:40 pee
12:00 pumped 7ml   2:47 fed (L)
1:55 fed (L)   3:03 fed (R)
2:10 fed (R) → 2:25 pooped/pee ?
2:40 expressed 12.5ml   = 33.5
4:10 fed (L)   3:10 pump 5cc
4:30 fed (R)   4:48 fed (L) x 10m
5:40 pump 10cc   5:15 pee/poo
6:04 poop/pee   5:20 fed (R) x 20m
6:10 fed (R)   5:50 pump 7cc
6:25 fed (L) x 10m
6:45 pump 12.5cc 7:40 pee
8:12 fed (L) x 10m 7:43 fed (L)
8:28 fed (R)   8:04 fed (R) fed/
9:00 pump 10cc   = 66cc → 8:30 poop
10:20 fed (L)   8:50 pump 30cc
10:40 fed (R)
10:57 pump 5cc
12:30 pee
12:40 fed (R) x 15m

DAY AND DATE: Tue Dec 27th (9a-9p)								
TIME	**START** (L or R)	**MINUTES** L	**MINUTES** R	**AMOUNT EXPRESSED**	**SUPPLEMENT AMOUNT** BREAST MILK	FORMULA	**OUTPUT** WET	POOP
1 10:00	R	17	13	@11:15 15cc			X	
2 12:15	R	14	15	@12:44 70cc	15ml		X	X
3 2:30	L	18	20	@2:10cc	1oz			
4 5:30	R	16	20	@5:73cc	90ml		X	X
5 8:00	L			@6:57 30cc			X	X
6 024t	R						X	X
7 9	R						X	X
8								
9								
10								
11								
12								
TOTALS:								

Six Days Old.

You are on a steep learning curve, and each day your baby changes. You may wonder when your baby will sleep longer at night or when she'll get on a schedule. It is normal to want some structure to your day; it's hard to be on call around the clock even for your beloved newborn (who may not seem so lovable at three in the morning!). Some babies adapt readily to feeding intervals of two to three hours, but most are unpredictable at this age. You may find that your baby will sleep if you hold her on your chest, but that if you lay her down she roots around as if she hasn't eaten at all!

For relief, have your partner calm and cuddle the baby as you nap, shower, or take a brisk walk. Keep up your strength by drinking plenty of fluids and eating high-energy foods.

The moment a child is born, the mother is also born.
She never existed before. The woman existed, but the mother,
never. A mother is something absolutely new.

—*Bhagwan Shree Rajneesh (Osho)*

7:20 pee
11:15 pump 15cc
12:44 " 10cc
7:00 pump 30cc

DAY AND DATE:

	TIME	START (L or R)	MINUTES L	R	AMOUNT EXPRESSED	SUPPLEMENT AMOUNT BREAST MILK	FORMULA	OUTPUT WET	POOP
1									
2									
3									
4									
5									
6									
7									
8									
9									
10									
11									
12									
TOTALS:									

One Week Old. Can you believe your baby has been in the world an entire week? While this week may seem like a blur, if you look how far you've come, and all the feedings you have logged and all the diapers you have changed, you will be impressed!

The first week is the "window" to initiate milk production, so this is the time to seek assistance if your breasts have not grown fuller or your baby has lost weight. Consistent milk removal—by nursing, pumping, or manual expression—is key if you find that your milk supply is lacking.

But perhaps instead you seem to have too much milk. If you are still uncomfortably engorged and leaking a lot, or if your baby is struggling to adapt to the fast flow, hang in there and, again, ask for help.

Absentmindedness begins in pregnancy but reaches its full and glorious bloom after the baby is born. You will come out of this fog. Write everything down.

—*Vicki Iovine*

9:00 15ml given
9:10 (L) ×10m
11:30 poop/pee
11:37 (R) ×15m
11:57 (L) ×10m →pump 30cc
1:20 poop/pee
1:27 (L) ×10m
1:52 (R) ×7m
2:00 90ml given
3:24 pump

DAY AND DATE: ....

	TIME	START (L or R)	MINUTES L	MINUTES R	AMOUNT EXPRESSED	SUPPLEMENT AMOUNT BREAST MILK	SUPPLEMENT AMOUNT FORMULA	OUTPUT WET	OUTPUT POOP
1									
2									
3									
4									
5									
6									
7									
8									
9									
10									
11									
12									
TOTALS:									

Eight Days Old.

As you begin the second week of your baby's life, you may wonder how you will be able to manage the baby's very time-consuming and sometimes overwhelming care. Perhaps your partner is returning to work, your relatives are leaving, or you have other children. Everyone may assume you will be running the household at full steam right away. But you are still recovering from the birth, learning the art of breastfeeding, and figuring out how to read your baby's cues. You need to decide what your priorities are and delegate as many household tasks as you can. There will be plenty of time to clean in the days to come.

Breastfeeding may or may not be getting easier. Feedings may take anywhere from 20 to 45 minutes. Your diary should show six to eight wet diapers and three or more stools bigger than a spoonful in each 24-hour period.

I was annoyed with my husband for not fully appreciating
how important and successful I was as a mother because
I'd kept both our daughter and myself alive for another day
and I hadn't burned down the house.

—*Debra Gilbert Rosenberg*

DAY AND DATE: ....

	TIME	START (L OR R)	MINUTES		AMOUNT EXPRESSED	SUPPLEMENT AMOUNT		OUTPUT	
			L	R		BREAST MILK	FORMULA	WET	POOP
1									
2									
3									
4									
5									
6									
7									
8									
9									
10									
11									
12									
		TOTALS:							

Nine Days Old.

Are you wondering when you should start pumping? Unless your baby can't latch on and suck well, you probably don't need to pump yet. In fact, a breast pump won't become necessary at all unless you are separated from your baby, you need to stimulate more milk production, or you want to skip a feeding so someone else can feed the baby. Other reasons women may pump are to relieve pronounced engorgement and to collect milk for later use.

If you need to pump to improve your milk production, or if your baby is premature or has other medical problems, rent a clinical-grade pump. Pump for about 10 minutes after feedings, and combine the small amounts you collect. You can offer this milk to the baby as needed or freeze it in 2- to 4-ounce portions. When you are expressing milk in lieu of a nursing session, pump for about 15 minutes.

After your milk supply is established, you can buy a retail pump, if you like. Before you purchase one, though, you'll want do some research, perhaps with the guidance of a lactation specialist. If breastfeeding is going well, you have plenty of time to begin this endeavor.

There are three reasons for breastfeeding: the milk is always at the right temperature; it comes in attractive containers; and the cat can't get it.

—*Irena Chalmers*

DAY AND DATE:

TIME	START (L or R)	MINUTES		AMOUNT EXPRESSED	SUPPLEMENT AMOUNT		OUTPUT	
		L	R		BREAST MILK	FORMULA	WET	POOP
1								
2								
3								
4								
5								
6								
7								
8								
9								
10								
11								
12								
TOTALS:								

10 Days Old. Just when you think your baby is getting more predictable, his nursing patterns may change. Feedings may cluster in the afternoon or evening, when your energy and patience may be at their lowest. If this happens, your baby is having an appetite spurt. So rock and roll with him! Nestle down in a comfortable place with a drink and snack nearby. Ask your partner for help when you need a break. Appetite spurts usually last only a few days, and then the milk supply increases and feedings even out again.

Mothers are basically a patient lot. They have to be or they would devour their offspring early on, like guppies.

—*Mary Daheim*

DAY AND DATE: ....

	TIME	START (L or R)	MINUTES L	R	AMOUNT EXPRESSED	SUPPLEMENT AMOUNT BREAST MILK	FORMULA	OUTPUT WET	POOP
1									
2									
3									
4									
5									
6									
7									
8									
9									
10									
11									
12									
TOTALS:									

11 Days Old.

At this point you may be wondering whether it's OK to introduce a pacifier or bottle.

It's common to offer a baby a pacifier to soothe her during a car ride or fussy spell or to help her get to sleep. But don't use a pacifier to delay feedings, because doing so could lead to early weaning.

Much ado is made about "nipple confusion," but a bigger problem with bottles is the fast flow of milk. If you elect to offer bottles during the first few weeks, use a slow-flow nipple, keep the baby semi-upright, and let her root for the nipple before you offer it. After your baby takes several swallows, lower the bottle and wait five to ten seconds before offering it again. Otherwise, your baby may gulp down the milk and still seem unsatisfied. If this happens, don't think it's because you aren't making enough milk. Also, be sure to express your milk in place of each bottle feeding.

6.13 @ 10ᵃᵐ

It's easy to know what a mother should do—until
you become one.

1:43 to 11:48
poop   pee
卌 +   卌 ll

—*Karen Lancaster Brown*

11:40-1:30 - sleep
1:76 (R) x 15m
1:48 (L) x 10m
12:10 pee
12:16 pee
2:30 - 3:30 sleep
3:30 (L) x 8m
3:59 (R) x 13m
4:15 - 5:05 sleep
5:10 poop/pee
5:23 (R) x 16m
5:42 (L) x 7m
5:45 - 7:30 sleep
:45 (L) x 14m ← 7:41 poop/pee
7:59 (R) x 8m
9:37 (R) x 11m
9:49 (L) x 76m
11:22 (R) x 9m
7:41 poop/pee
9:45 ''

DAY AND DATE: ....

	TIME	START (L or R)	MINUTES L	MINUTES R	AMOUNT EXPRESSED	SUPPLEMENT AMOUNT BREAST MILK	SUPPLEMENT AMOUNT FORMULA	OUTPUT WET	OUTPUT POOP
1									
2									
3									
4									
5									
6									
7									
8									
9									
10									
11									
12									
TOTALS:									

12 Days Old. Are you concerned about your baby's gas and hiccups? Because of babies' immature digestive tracts, a lot of gas and hiccups is usually normal.

To minimize gas attacks, give the baby a chance to burp after nursing at each breast, by sitting him up or laying him over your shoulder. If your baby is fussy between feedings, pressure and warmth may comfort him. Try swaddling him lightly in a light blanket, or let him rest on his stomach over your lap or arm.

Baby: An alimentary canal with a loud voice at one end and no responsibility at the other.

—*Elizabeth Adamson*

11-12:50 sleep
12:50-1:00 (R)
1-1:11 (L)
1:15-3:33 sleep
3:35-3:48 (L)
3:55 (R) x 11m
4 (R) x 17m
6:18 (L) x 16m
7:30- sleep

DAY AND DATE: . . . .

	TIME	START (L or R)	MINUTES L	R	AMOUNT EXPRESSED	SUPPLEMENT AMOUNT BREAST MILK	FORMULA	OUTPUT WET	POOP
1									
2									
3									
4									
5									
6									
7									
8									
9									
10									
11									
12									
TOTALS:									

13 Days Old. Your baby's doctor may have scheduled a visit for about this time to check your baby's weight gain and to answer any questions you may have. If all is well, your baby will have regained her birth weight and will be gaining an ounce a day. This should assure you that you have established a good milk supply. Continue nursing every two to three hours during the day, but don't wake the baby for night feedings if she is back to her birth weight. As long as you are nursing at least eight times in every twenty-four hours, it's fine for your baby to sleep a four- to five-hour stretch at night—and heavenly for you!

If you are still battling sore nipples, or if your baby is having trouble latching on or is gaining poorly, it's vital to find support and guidance. Ask your doctor for a referral to a lactation consultant, or call your local La Leche League.

If your baby is "beautiful and perfect, never cries or fusses, sleeps on schedule and burps on demand, an angel all the time," you're the grandma.

—Teresa Bloomingdale

DAY AND DATE:..

	TIME	START (L or R)	MINUTES L	MINUTES R	AMOUNT EXPRESSED	SUPPLEMENT AMOUNT BREAST MILK	SUPPLEMENT AMOUNT FORMULA	OUTPUT WET	OUTPUT POOP
1									
2									
3									
4									
5									
6									
7									
8									
9									
10									
11									
12									
	TOTALS:								

Two Weeks Old. Can you believe your little one has been here for two weeks? Your world may seem to consist of nothing but feedings, diaper changes, laundry, and fatigue.

Find creative ways to grab naps. If you haven't already, learn to nurse lying down.

If friends and family members ask what you need, take all the help you can get. Let someone stay with the baby while you go outdoors or take a long afternoon nap.

As your friends may tell you, the first couple of weeks after birth are the toughest. You have survived. Give yourself a pat on the back, and admire the baby you are nourishing and nurturing!

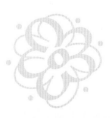

Your baby will not only survive your mothering; he will thrive
and live to be your lord and master.

—*Vicki Iovine*

DAY AND DATE: ....

	TIME	START (L or R)	MINUTES L	R	AMOUNT EXPRESSED	SUPPLEMENT AMOUNT BREAST MILK	FORMULA	OUTPUT WET	POOP
1									
2									
3									
4									
5									
6									
7									
8									
9									
10									
11									
12									
TOTALS:									

15 Days Old. If your baby was born at 37 weeks gestation or earlier, he may be finally nearing his due date. You have probably been expressing your milk to make up for his lack of stamina at the breast, and he may still be in the hospital. At this point you may be able to offer the breast with more regularity; ask for help. When he is discharged, get advice on providing supplementary feedings until he is able to get all his nourishment at the breast (if the baby has medical problems, a lactation specialist's guidance is essential). Keep up your milk supply by expressing for a few minutes after each nursing. Use this diary to chart intake and output. An early baby can be a challenge, but most preemies will eventually take all their milk at the breast.

A baby is a question mark and his mother is the answer he seeks.
Sensitive to every new encounter, the newborn experiences life
through the soft filter of his mother's embrace, her milk, her
lullabies. He recognizes you by sight and by touch—you sense
his needs and his separate self. Together you will learn.

—*Deborah Jackson*

DAY AND DATE: ....

	TIME	START (L or R)	MINUTES L	MINUTES R	AMOUNT EXPRESSED	SUPPLEMENT AMOUNT BREAST MILK	SUPPLEMENT AMOUNT FORMULA	OUTPUT WET	OUTPUT POOP
1									
2									
3									
4									
5									
6									
7									
8									
9									
10									
11									
12									
TOTALS:									

16 Days Old.

Do you feel lost in a maze of feedings and baby care? Try to shower and dress before the day unravels. Plan just one activity you can finish today.

If you have left home only for doctor's appointments and quick errands, you have probably developed a case of cabin fever. Take a break to do something for you. Invite a friend over, and have her bring lunch. Or get out of the house for a walk or just a sit on the porch. Perhaps someone can drive you on a few errands and wait in the car with the baby. Anything that connects to your former life will help you feel better during this period.

Cleaning your house while your kids are still growing is like shoveling the walk before it stops snowing.

—*Phyllis Diller*

_____

_____

_____

_____

_____

_____

_____

_____

_____

_____

_____

_____

_____

_____

_____

_____

_____

_____

_____

_____

DAY AND **DATE**:

	TIME	START (L OR R)	MINUTES L	R	AMOUNT EXPRESSED	SUPPLEMENT AMOUNT BREAST MILK	FORMULA	OUTPUT WET	POOP
1									
2									
3									
4									
5									
6									
7									
8									
9									
10									
11									
12									
TOTALS:									

17 Days Old. Some mothers find that, for any of a multitude of reasons, they end up pumping for most or all of the baby's feedings. If this happens to you, you are taking on a labor of love. Make it easier by using an effective electric pump that allows you to pump from both breasts at once. This way you'll collect the most milk in the least amount of time. Consider investing in a special bra that lets you pump hands-free, so you can do other things while you're pumping. For optimal milk production, pump about eight times in each twenty-four hours, including at least once in the night. Congratulate yourself on providing breast milk for your little one, no matter how much or for how long.

The most important thing she'd learned over the years was that there was no way to be a perfect mother and a million ways to be a good one.

—*Jill Churchill*

DAY AND DATE: ....

	TIME	START (L or R)	MINUTES L	R	AMOUNT EXPRESSED	SUPPLEMENT AMOUNT BREAST MILK	FORMULA	OUTPUT WET	POOP
1									
2									
3									
4									
5									
6									
7									
8									
9									
10									
11									
12									
TOTALS:									

18 Days Old. By this time, your baby may be wakeful and active, especially from late afternoon until late at night. If she fusses a lot in the evening, she may be needing to nurse more often to increase your milk supply, or she may simply be overtired.

You may wonder if something you are eating could be causing your baby's distress. Most breastfeeding mothers can eat as they normally do without upsetting their babies. Many mothers suspect a link, however, between their babies' fussiness and foods in their own diet. These foods may include gas-producing vegetables (such as cabbage), chocolate, citrus fruits and their juices, and spicy foods. If your baby gets fussy and spits up a lot two to six hours after you eat one of these foods, try omitting it from your diet.

Dairy products, in either the mother's diet or in formula, sometimes cause spitting up, congestion, and watery, green stools. The stools may also be mucous or even streaked with blood. If you see these symptoms, consult your baby's doctor. You may need to eliminate all dairy products from your diet.

Motherhood has a very humanizing effect. Everything gets reduced to essentials.

—*Meryl Streep*

DAY and DATE: ....

	TIME	START (L or R)	MINUTES L	MINUTES R	AMOUNT EXPRESSED	SUPPLEMENT AMOUNT BREAST MILK	SUPPLEMENT AMOUNT FORMULA	OUTPUT WET	OUTPUT POOP
1									
2									
3									
4									
5									
6									
7									
8									
9									
10									
11									
12									
	TOTALS:								

19 Days Old.

It's time to take your emotional temperature. If you are experiencing racing thoughts, uncontrollable crying jags, feelings of worthlessness, lack of appetite, insomnia, or even fears of hurting your baby, you need to discuss theses feelings with your doctor. Women who have suffered severe depression or anxiety in the past sometimes find these feelings resurfacing in the weeks after giving birth. Fatigue and fluctuating hormones may bring on the symptoms. New research suggests that supplements of long-chain Omega-3 fatty acids may help with postpartum depression. In some cases medication is needed; fortunately, most of the drugs are compatible with breastfeeding. In any case, if you're feeling very depressed or anxious you should not suffer in silence. Only by caring for yourself can you care for your baby.

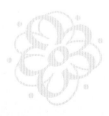

Motherhood brings as much joy as ever, but it still brings boredom, exhaustion, and sorrow too. Nothing else will ever make you as happy or as sad, as proud or as tired, for nothing is quite as hard as helping a person develop his own individuality—especially while you struggle to keep your own.

—*Marguerite Kelly and Elia Parsons*

DAY AND DATE:

	TIME	START (L or R)	MINUTES L	MINUTES R	AMOUNT EXPRESSED	SUPPLEMENT AMOUNT BREAST MILK	SUPPLEMENT AMOUNT FORMULA	OUTPUT WET	OUTPUT POOP
1									
2									
3									
4									
5									
6									
7									
8									
9									
10									
11									
12									
TOTALS:									

20 Days Old.

Your baby is nearly three weeks old now. He is probably awake more than before, and for unpredictable intervals. Instead of trying to divide your life between baby-time and you-time, try going about your daily tasks while wearing your baby in a sling or wrap. Your baby will love the motion and being close to you, and you will be able to enjoy his new alertness and soothe him as needed while doing other things. You may feel less stressed about "doing it all" when you do it with your baby in tow!

If evolution really works, how come mothers only
have two hands?

—*Ed Dussault*

_____
_____
_____
_____
_____
_____
_____
_____
_____
_____
_____
_____
_____
_____
_____
_____
_____
_____
_____
_____
_____

DAY AND DATE: ....

	TIME	START (L or R)	MINUTES L	MINUTES R	AMOUNT EXPRESSED	SUPPLEMENT AMOUNT BREAST MILK	SUPPLEMENT AMOUNT FORMULA	OUTPUT WET	OUTPUT POOP
1									
2									
3									
4									
5									
6									
7									
8									
9									
10									
11									
12									
TOTALS:									

Three Weeks Old. Week Three is a pivotal time in your baby's development. If she was born at full term, she should be able to latch on to your breast easily now. She is more alert and engaged with the world, and she is likely to alternate between contentment and episodes of fussiness and frequent nursing. Another appetite spurt may occur at this time, and you may doubt your milk supply as your nursling embarks on another feeding marathon. Go with the flow, and look at your diary to see how far you have come!

Babies are always more trouble than you thought—
and more wonderful.

—Charles Osgood

DAY and DATE: ....

	TIME	START (L or R)	MINUTES L	MINUTES R	AMOUNT EXPRESSED	SUPPLEMENT AMOUNT BREAST MILK	SUPPLEMENT AMOUNT FORMULA	OUTPUT WET	OUTPUT POOP
1									
2									
3									
4									
5									
6									
7									
8									
9									
10									
11									
12									
TOTALS:									

22 Days Old. At this point sore nipples should be a thing of the past. If your nipples have been sore all along, or if they suddenly start hurting, get help. After the first few weeks of nursing, continued nipple soreness may be caused by dermatitis, infection, or vasospasm. If your nipples suddenly start hurting, a yeast infection may be the cause. A lactation specialist can identify these conditions, and a doctor can provide treatment as needed. Don't let sore nipples take the pleasure out of nursing!

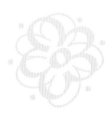

I make milk; what's your superpower?

—*Heather Cushman-Dowdee*

DAY AND DATE: . . . .

| | TIME | START (L or R) | MINUTES | | AMOUNT EXPRESSED | SUPPLEMENT AMOUNT | | OUTPUT | |
			L	R		BREAST MILK	FORMULA	WET	POOP
1									
2									
3									
4									
5									
6									
7									
8									
9									
10									
11									
12									
TOTALS:									

23 Days Old.

After the first three weeks, many babies have long, regular episodes of inconsolable crying. This is called *colic*—a word that strikes fear in the hearts of new parents.

In some cases the problem is reflux, which just means spitting up. All babies spit up, but some experience pain from the backwash of acidic milk into the esophagus. If your baby has colicky crying episodes, if he arches his back and pulls off the breast during feedings, if he resists lying flat and roots for the breast after feedings, and if he is generally unhappy, reflux may be the problem.

Some colicky babies seem to suffer with gas and cramps. A certain food in the mother's diet can be the culprit, so keeping track of what you eat may help if your baby has colic. If you have an abundant supply of milk, your baby may be taking a disproportionate amount of the low-fat milk produced early in the feeding, especially if you switch him to the other side before the first breast is fully drained. You may need to limit the baby to one breast per feeding.

If your baby is colicky, enlist help during trying times of the day. Write in your diary when the episodes occur, and make other notes about the baby's behavior. Your observations will enable your lactation specialist or doctor to help you identify the problem.

Here's the truth: The birth of a baby is supposed to blow your schedule to bits, even if it nearly kills you and your partner. This is nature's way of making sure that we get our new priorities straight. The three most important become, in this order: (1) the baby's health, (2) the baby's comfort, and (3) the baby's parents' survival. (This is a very distant third.)

—*Vicki Iovine*

DAY and DATE: ....

	TIME	START (L or R)	MINUTES L	MINUTES R	AMOUNT EXPRESSED	SUPPLEMENT AMOUNT BREAST MILK	SUPPLEMENT AMOUNT FORMULA	OUTPUT WET	OUTPUT POOP
1									
2									
3									
4									
5									
6									
7									
8									
9									
10									
11									
12									
TOTALS:									

24 Days Old.

Overabundant milk can make both mother and baby uncomfortable. If you have this problem, your breasts may feel overfull. They may leak constantly and never soften, and you may be at increased risk for plugged ducts and even breast infections. Your milk may spray forcefully, causing the baby to lose suction, sputter, cough, or gulp during feedings. Your baby may have excess gas and hiccups and explosive, watery stools.

The key to taming this problem is to reduce milk production. Start by offering just one breast for most of the feeding, or even the entire feeding. This will leave the other breast overly full until the next feeding, so initially you may need to express a little milk to relieve a bit of the pressure. A lactation specialist can help you figure out what works best for you and your baby.

To the whole world you might be just one person, but to one person you might just be the whole world.

—*Joseph Campbell*

_____

_____

_____

_____

_____

_____

_____

_____

_____

_____

_____

_____

_____

_____

_____

_____

_____

_____

_____

DAY AND DATE:

	TIME	START (L or R)	MINUTES L	MINUTES R	AMOUNT EXPRESSED	SUPPLEMENT AMOUNT BREAST MILK	SUPPLEMENT AMOUNT FORMULA	OUTPUT WET	OUTPUT POOP
1									
2									
3									
4									
5									
6									
7									
8									
9									
10									
11									
12									
TOTALS:									

25 Days Old. Are you and your partner bickering over things that would not ordinarily bother you? You are both undergoing a huge, life-changing event as you settle in to your new roles as parents. Perhaps a date night at home would be a nice distraction from the daily whirlwind. If your partner has felt left out, this could be a way to give him some attention—even though the best-laid plans can be interrupted by a crying baby. How about a picnic with take-out on the living room floor, followed by a movie or favorite TV show? You may have to take turns eating, but at least you will be together, even if you're eating fast food in front of the TV. Let your partner know how much his support means to you.

With all the attention paid to your new baby, it is easy for your own feelings and needs to get lost in the shuffle. Although all parents engage in some self-sacrifice for their children, keep in mind that your goal isn't just to raise a happy, healthy child. You want that child to be part of a happy, healthy family as well.

—*Lawrence Kutner*

DAY AND DATE: ....

	TIME	START (L or R)	MINUTES L	MINUTES R	AMOUNT EXPRESSED	SUPPLEMENT AMOUNT BREAST MILK	SUPPLEMENT AMOUNT FORMULA	OUTPUT WET	OUTPUT POOP
1									
2									
3									
4									
5									
6									
7									
8									
9									
10									
11									
12									
TOTALS:									

26 Days Old. Now that you are feeling more confident in your mothering abilities, unsolicited advice from others may sting. Most folks think they are being helpful when they share nuggets of parenting wisdom, but you may feel they are criticizing you or doubting your capabilities. It may be especially hard when someone wonders if your baby is "getting enough to eat" or suggests that you give the baby a bottle. The best tack may be to remain silent and nod or to give a pat answer like "Thanks, I'll consider that," while biting your tongue.

Don't let unsolicited advice shake your confidence. You are the expert on your baby.

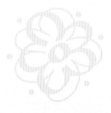

What good mothers and fathers instinctively feel like doing
for their babies is usually best after all.

—Benjamin Spock

_____

_____

_____

_____

_____

_____

_____

_____

_____

_____

_____

_____

_____

_____

_____

_____

_____

_____

DAY AND DATE: . . . .

	TIME	START (L or R)	MINUTES L	MINUTES R	AMOUNT EXPRESSED	SUPPLEMENT AMOUNT BREAST MILK	SUPPLEMENT AMOUNT FORMULA	OUTPUT WET	OUTPUT POOP
1									
2									
3									
4									
5									
6									
7									
8									
9									
10									
11									
12									
TOTALS:									

27 Days Old. Now that nursing is probably natural and effortless for you, you can begin planning for times when you will miss a feeding. To start collecting milk for someone else to feed the baby, practice hand expression, or, to save time, select a breast pump that will allow pumping from both breasts at once. Beware, though: Not all pumps are created equal; they come in a variety of models and prices, and the prices don't always reflect quality. Do some research to determine which model will best serve your purposes. *The Nursing Mother's Companion, Sixth Edition,* has a large section devoted to pump selection.

Being a full-time mother is one of the highest salaried jobs,
since the payment is pure love.

—*Mildred B. Vermont*

DAY and DATE: ....

	TIME	START (L or R)	MINUTES L	MINUTES R	AMOUNT EXPRESSED	SUPPLEMENT AMOUNT BREAST MILK	SUPPLEMENT AMOUNT FORMULA	OUTPUT WET	OUTPUT POOP
1									
2									
3									
4									
5									
6									
7									
8									
9									
10									
11									
12									
TOTALS:									

28 Days Old. After you select a pump, your next task is to learn about the safe storage of breast milk. When pumping and handling your milk, first make sure your hands, pump parts, and containers are clean. Keep your milk in the refrigerator if you plan to use it in within three days; otherwise store it in the freezer. See *The Nursing Mother's Companion* for complete guidelines on storing and thawing breast milk and preparing bottles.

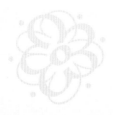

Breastfeeding is a mother's gift to herself, her baby,
and the earth.

—Pamela K. Wiggins

_____

_____

_____

_____

_____

_____

_____

_____

_____

_____

_____

_____

_____

_____

_____

_____

_____

_____

_____

DAY AND DATE:

	TIME	START (L OR R)	MINUTES L	MINUTES R	AMOUNT EXPRESSED	SUPPLEMENT AMOUNT BREAST MILK	SUPPLEMENT AMOUNT FORMULA	OUTPUT WET	OUTPUT POOP
1									
2									
3									
4									
5									
6									
7									
8									
9									
10									
11									
12									
TOTALS:									

29 Days Old. If you plan to have Dad or someone else feed the baby when you're away but you haven't introduced a bottle yet, this is the time to do it. Some babies resist the bottle if it isn't offered during the first month or so.

Offer the bottle soon after you have breastfed the baby, so she isn't frantic with hunger. Better yet, have someone else offer the bottle while you're out on a short errand. Provide just an ounce or two of milk. Once the baby accepts the bottle, she should continue to do so if you offer it every couple of days. Bottle feeding your breast milk won't threaten your supply provided you express your milk at about the time of each bottle feeding.

In the sheltered simplicity of the first days after a baby is born, one sees again the magical closed circle, the miraculous sense of two people existing only for each other.

—Anne Morrow Lindbergh

_____

_____

_____

_____

_____

_____

_____

_____

_____

_____

_____

_____

_____

_____

_____

_____

_____

_____

_____

DAY AND DATE:..

	TIME	START (L or R)	MINUTES L	MINUTES R	AMOUNT EXPRESSED	SUPPLEMENT AMOUNT BREAST MILK	SUPPLEMENT AMOUNT FORMULA	OUTPUT WET	OUTPUT POOP
1									
2									
3									
4									
5									
6									
7									
8									
9									
10									
11									
12									
TOTALS:									

One Month Old. At the end of your baby's first month, your new-born is becoming his own little person. You are better able to discern his cues and find ways to meet his many needs. Your diary will reflect the effort you have put into getting started with breastfeeding.

You will be seeing the baby's doctor for a one-month checkup soon. List your questions and concerns here, and take them along to the appointment. During the visit, you can record the baby's weight, length, and growth percentiles in your diary.

Congratulations on reaching this milestone!

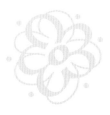

This [new] period of parenting is an intense one. Never will we know such responsibility, such productive and hard work, such potential for isolation in the caretaking role and such intimacy and close involvement in the growth and development of another human being.

—*Joan Sheingold Ditzion*

DAY AND DATE:

	TIME	START (L or R)	MINUTES L	R	AMOUNT EXPRESSED	SUPPLEMENT AMOUNT BREAST MILK	FORMULA	OUTPUT WET	POOP
1									
2									
3									
4									
5									
6									
7									
8									
9									
10									
11									
12									
TOTALS:									

31 Days Old. As breastfeeding becomes second nature and you get back in the swing of things beyond your home, you may feel you have one foot in the nursery and one foot ready to step back into your life as it was before you gave birth. You are a new person now; motherhood is part of your identity. You may at once see yourself as "only a mother," struggling to protect your time with your baby, and simultaneously yearn to reclaim aspects of your pre-baby lifestyle. This confusion is common to all new mothers. Reflecting on all you have experienced this last month, and your accomplishments in general, will help you integrate your new persona. Be patient with yourself.

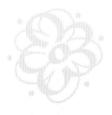

A hundred years from now, it will not matter what my bank account was, the sort of house I lived in, or the kind of car I drove, but the world may be different because I was important in the life of a child.

—*Kathy Davis*

DAY AND DATE:

	TIME	START (L or R)	MINUTES L	MINUTES R	AMOUNT EXPRESSED	SUPPLEMENT AMOUNT BREAST MILK	SUPPLEMENT AMOUNT FORMULA	OUTPUT WET	OUTPUT POOP
1									
2									
3									
4									
5									
6									
7									
8									
9									
10									
11									
12									
			TOTALS:						

32 Days Old. You may no longer find it necessary to record the details of every feeding and diaper change. But you might keep track of the number of daily feedings, note if you offer a top-off after nursing or supplement a feeding for a nursing session, and record how much milk you express, if you are expressing at all. You should still expect a minimum of eight feedings in every twenty-four hours. Dropping below eight feedings at this time could result in lower milk production and less weight gain for your baby.

You will be glad you kept this permanent record of your sweet baby's days.

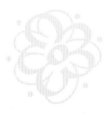

Sometimes the laughter in mothering is the recognition of the ironies and absurdities. Sometimes, though, it's just pure, unthinkable delight.

—*Barbara Schapiro*

DAY and DATE: ....

	TIME	START (L or R)	MINUTES L	MINUTES R	AMOUNT EXPRESSED	SUPPLEMENT AMOUNT BREAST MILK	SUPPLEMENT AMOUNT FORMULA	OUTPUT WET	OUTPUT POOP
1									
2									
3									
4									
5									
6									
7									
8									
9									
10									
11									
12									
TOTALS:									

33 Days Old. If you think you will never get a full night's sleep again, you are wrong. But it may be a while. In the meantime, find creative ways to get more sleep. During the day, turn off the phones and take a nap. Nurse lying down so you can relax and doze. When your partner comes home, hand him the baby as you greet him, and then sneak off for a warm shower and a short nap before joining him for a late dinner.

At night, it will help to keep the baby near you, in a bassinet, a baby bed affixed to your own (such as a Co-Sleeper), or a baby bed that you set on top of your own (such as a Snuggle Nest). This way you won't have to take a walk to nurse the baby, and Dad can easily do the burping, changing, and resettling. Someday you will sleep through the night once more!

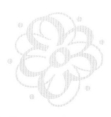

There never was a child so lovely but his mother was glad
to get him asleep.

—Ralph Waldo Emerson

_____

_____

_____

_____

_____

_____

_____

_____

_____

_____

_____

_____

_____

_____

_____

_____

_____

_____

_____

_____

_____

_____

DAY and DATE: ....

	TIME	START (L or R)	MINUTES L	MINUTES R	AMOUNT EXPRESSED	SUPPLEMENT AMOUNT BREAST MILK	SUPPLEMENT AMOUNT FORMULA	OUTPUT WET	OUTPUT POOP
1									
2									
3									
4									
5									
6									
7									
8									
9									
10									
11									
12									
TOTALS:									

34 Days Old. At this point you are probably longing to get out of the house more. Maybe your doctor has told you to postpone exercising, or maybe the baby's doctor has told you to avoid crowds. If so, you should soon get the go-ahead for socializing, exercise, and even sex. Think about what you'd like to do with the baby in tow. Take an infant massage class? Have lunch with friends? Start attending meetings of La Leche League or another moms' group? Make plans for something you can look forward to, even if it is just a trip to the local coffee shop.

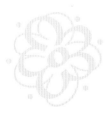

Believe it or not, today offers you a hidden gift, if you're
willing to search for it.

—Sarah Ban Breathnach

_____

_____

_____

_____

_____

_____

_____

_____

_____

_____

_____

_____

_____

_____

_____

_____

_____

_____

DAY AND DATE:...

	TIME	START (L or R)	MINUTES L	MINUTES R	AMOUNT EXPRESSED	SUPPLEMENT AMOUNT BREAST MILK	SUPPLEMENT AMOUNT FORMULA	OUTPUT WET	OUTPUT POOP
1									
2									
3									
4									
5									
6									
7									
8									
9									
10									
11									
12									
	TOTALS:								

35 Days Old. Now that the size of your breasts has settled, this may be the time to purchase a few nursing bras. Not only are good nursing bras supportive and comfortable, but they have cup flaps for easy access to the breasts. Find a store with a clerk who is proficient at fitting nursing mothers; as with regular bras, getting a good fit is worth any extra time and money required.

Those elastic-waist pants may still be a staple in your wardrobe, but don't despair; it took nine months to put on the extra weight, and you will shed the pounds slowly but surely while nursing. Update your look with some scarves and roomy tops until you are back in your skinny jeans.

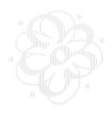

Nursing does not diminish the beauty of a woman's breasts;
it enhances their charm by making them look lived in
and happy.

— *Robert A. Heinlein*

_____

_____

_____

_____

_____

_____

_____

_____

_____

_____

_____

_____

_____

_____

_____

_____

_____

_____

DAY and DATE:

	TIME	START (L or R)	MINUTES L	MINUTES R	AMOUNT EXPRESSED	SUPPLEMENT AMOUNT BREAST MILK	SUPPLEMENT AMOUNT FORMULA	OUTPUT WET	OUTPUT POOP
1									
2									
3									
4									
5									
6									
7									
8									
9									
10									
11									
12									
TOTALS:									

36 Days Old.
Are you wishing for the company and support of other nursing mothers? Attending a La Leche League meeting is a wonderful way to get it. La Leche League International is an organization that "helps mothers worldwide to breastfeed through mother-to-mother support, encouragement, information, and education," and promotes "a better understanding of breast-feeding as an important element in the healthy development of the baby and mother." Most communities have a La Leche League chapter; your lactation specialist or childbirth educator can refer you to one, or to another local group or class for new mothers. For more information, see the website at www.llli.org.

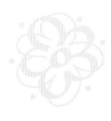

You see, it isn't that you aren't interesting anymore,
it is simply that what interests you is deep and narrow
and consuming.

—*Debra Gilbert Rosenberg*

DAY and DATE: ....

TIME	START (L or R)	MINUTES		AMOUNT EXPRESSED	SUPPLEMENT AMOUNT		OUTPUT	
		L	R		BREAST MILK	FORMULA	WET	POOP
1								
2								
3								
4								
5								
6								
7								
8								
9								
10								
11								
12								
TOTALS:								

37 Days Old. Although breastfed babies are much more portable than bottle-fed ones, it takes planning to get yourself, the baby, and your gear together and to your destination in a reasonable amount of time. Pack just one bag or backpack with your wallet and essential baby items. Leave out anything that you won't actually use while you're out. Keep extra supplies—diapers, changing pad, wipes, and baby clothes—in your car at all times. Nurse just before you leave home so you can get where you're going before nursing again. If you're going shopping, try to pick up as many things you need as possible in the same shopping center or neighborhood so you can avoid getting in and out of the car repeatedly. While you're walking, you will find that having the baby in a sling or stroller is easier than carrying the baby around in a car seat.

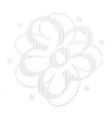

When you are a mother, you are never really alone in your thoughts. A mother always has to think twice, once for herself and once for her child.

—*Sophia Loren*

DAY and DATE:...

	TIME	START (L or R)	MINUTES L	MINUTES R	AMOUNT EXPRESSED	SUPPLEMENT AMOUNT BREAST MILK	SUPPLEMENT AMOUNT FORMULA	OUTPUT WET	OUTPUT POOP
1									
2									
3									
4									
5									
6									
7									
8									
9									
10									
11									
12									
			TOTALS:						

38 Days Old.

Adding a third person can strain a household to a degree few couples expect. Sleep deprivation and baby care devour the time and energy you and your partner used to reserve for each other. Fatigue, daily frustrations, and poor communication breed resentments on both sides. You want Dad to do more, but he wonders why you get nothing done all day.

Remember, you and the baby have formed a circle that often closes Dad out. Invite him in, and not only when the baby is fussy. Avoid criticizing your partner's attempts at bathing, soothing, or diapering, even if he puts the diaper on backward. Like you, he will learn along the way. He and the baby will form their own special bond, if you let them.

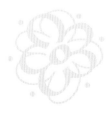

Having a child is surely the most beautifully irrational
act that two people in love can commit.

—*Bill Cosby*

_____

_____

_____

_____

_____

_____

_____

_____

_____

_____

_____

_____

_____

_____

_____

_____

_____

_____

DAY AND DATE: . . . .

	TIME	START (L or R)	MINUTES L	MINUTES R	AMOUNT EXPRESSED	SUPPLEMENT AMOUNT BREAST MILK	SUPPLEMENT AMOUNT FORMULA	OUTPUT WET	OUTPUT POOP
1									
2									
3									
4									
5									
6									
7									
8									
9									
10									
11									
12									
TOTALS:									

39 Days Old. You may be surprised to find that your baby is having fewer bowel movements after the first month. So long as your baby is gaining weight well, a drop in the daily diaper count is normal; it doesn't mean your baby is constipated or underfed. Expect continued daily weight gains of about an ounce per day for the next couple of months. Bowel movement should still be loose; you shouldn't see formed stools until the baby begins eating solid foods.

You may occasionally notice greenish bowel movements, but unless you see mucus or blood this shouldn't worry you.

If you have an oversupply of milk, your baby may ingest too much foremilk and react with very watery bowel movements. In this case, be sure you're draining one breast completely before switching the baby to the other side.

If you are concerned about any changes in your baby's urine or bowel movements, consult the baby's doctor.

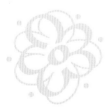

A baby changes your dinner party conversation from
politics to poops.

—*Maurice Johnstone*

_____

_____

_____

_____

_____

_____

_____

_____

_____

_____

_____

_____

_____

_____

_____

_____

_____

_____

_____

_____

DAY AND DATE: ....

	TIME	START (L or R)	MINUTES L	MINUTES R	AMOUNT EXPRESSED	SUPPLEMENT AMOUNT BREAST MILK	SUPPLEMENT AMOUNT FORMULA	OUTPUT WET	OUTPUT POOP
1									
2									
3									
4									
5									
6									
7									
8									
9									
10									
11									
12									
TOTALS:									

40 Days Old. Your midwife or doctor has probably asked you to schedule an appointment for four to six weeks after your baby's birth. You can expect to talk about resuming both intercourse and contraception. Breastfeeding by itself is an effective form of contraception during the first six months post partum, if you are nursing or expressing frequently around the clock. If you go long intervals at night without feeding, or if you fail to express when someone else feeds the baby formula, your fertility may resume early.

If you elect to use another form of contraception, be careful with hormonal products. Oral, vaginal, injectable, and intrauterine contraceptives are suitable for nursing mothers provided they are free of estrogen. Even small amounts of estrogen can decrease milk production.

List questions for your doctor or midwife in this diary, and bring it to the appointment so you'll be sure to address all your concerns.

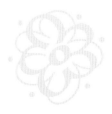

I didn't know how babies were made until I was
pregnant with my fourth child.

—*Loretta Lynn*

DAY AND DATE: ....

	TIME	START (L or R)	MINUTES L	MINUTES R	AMOUNT EXPRESSED	SUPPLEMENT AMOUNT BREAST MILK	SUPPLEMENT AMOUNT FORMULA	OUTPUT WET	OUTPUT POOP
1									
2									
3									
4									
5									
6									
7									
8									
9									
10									
11									
12									
			TOTALS:						

41 Days Old. If you have been craving some vigorous physical activity, you may wonder if exercising could affect the supply or composition of your breast milk. Although exercising doesn't affect a mother's milk supply, it can slightly increase the amount of lactic acid in the milk. Still, your baby will enjoy nursing as much after you exercise as before, and she won't even mind if your are sweaty!

You will want to follow several guidelines when you resume exercising. First, try to nurse just prior to vigorous exercising, so your breasts will be lighter. Wear a supportive bra; if you are large-breasted, you may need to wear two jogging bras. Drink plenty of fluids. Brisk walking is fine, and it allows you to take the baby along. Working out at a gym is all right, too. Whatever sort of exercise you choose, start slowly and work up to your previous level of exertion. You will end up a revitalized mother.

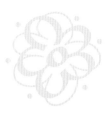

I do yoga and Pilates, but the body itself knows what
to do. When you're breastfeeding, the body has its own
way to shrink.

—*Toni Collette*

DAY AND DATE: ....

	TIME	START (L OR R)	MINUTES L	MINUTES R	AMOUNT EXPRESSED	SUPPLEMENT AMOUNT BREAST MILK	SUPPLEMENT AMOUNT FORMULA	OUTPUT WET	OUTPUT POOP
1									
2									
3									
4									
5									
6									
7									
8									
9									
10									
11									
12									
TOTALS:									

42 Days Old. Concerns about body image seem universal among women and are certainly prevalent in the postpartum period. For many mothers, the remaining weight gained during pregnancy is a source of distress.

You'd be unrealistic to expect to bounce back to your normal weight and size by six weeks after giving birth. But the extra calories you spend to produce milk should help bring slow, steady weight loss. Quick-weight-loss plans are not a good idea when you're nursing, but many well-known weight-loss groups have sensible programs geared to lactating mothers. Keep energy bars and fruits and veggies within reach when you are stressed, because fatigue and stress tend to diminish resistance to unhealthy snacks.

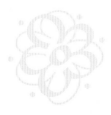

It took nine months to gain the weight, and it will probably take nine months to take it off.

—*Vicki Iovine*

_____

_____

_____

_____

_____

_____

_____

_____

_____

_____

_____

_____

_____

_____

_____

_____

_____

_____

DAY AND DATE: ....

	TIME	START (L or R)	MINUTES L	R	AMOUNT EXPRESSED	SUPPLEMENT AMOUNT BREAST MILK	FORMULA	OUTPUT WET	POOP
1									
2									
3									
4									
5									
6									
7									
8									
9									
10									
11									
12									
TOTALS:									

43 Days Old. If your baby hasn't yet rewarded you with her first smiles, you will soon be captivated with them. At first you may think, Was that really a smile? Or was it only gas? But then you'll get another smile, and your heart will melt. You'll find that your baby is quite a sociable little creature, when she isn't burping, spitting up, passing gas, or pooping.

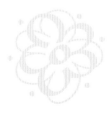

The baby has learned to smile, and her smiles burst forth like holiday sparklers, lighting our hearts.

Joy fills the room. At what are we smiling? We don't know, we don't care. We are communicating with one another in happiness, and the smiles are the outward display of our delight and our love.

—*Joan Lowery Nixon*

_____

_____

_____

_____

_____

_____

_____

_____

_____

_____

_____

_____

_____

_____

_____

_____

_____

_____

DAY AND DATE: ....

	TIME	START (L or R)	MINUTES		AMOUNT EXPRESSED	SUPPLEMENT AMOUNT		OUTPUT	
			L	R		BREAST MILK	FORMULA	WET	POOP
1									
2									
3									
4									
5									
6									
7									
8									
9									
10									
11									
12									
TOTALS:									

44 Days Old. At your baby's one-month checkup, the doctor may have mentioned the importance of "tummy time." Because we no longer place babies on their stomachs to sleep, and because many, unfortunately, spend a great deal of time in car seats, infant carriers, and swings, face-down play time provides valuable exercise to strengthen the baby's neck, shoulder, and head muscles and helps ensure a rounded head shape. Tummy time is also an opportunity to play with your baby.

To start, place the baby on a blanket on the floor, face down, and talk to him and stroke him. Don't be surprised if he objects at first. You can start out doing this for just a few minutes at a time and slowly build up to ten minutes or more several times a day. Dad can join in this endeavor, too. With consistency, you will find that your baby begins to enjoy the play, and you'll see progress in his development as he raises his head with ease, turning from side to side.

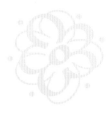

Babies need social interactions with loving adults who talk with them, listen to their babblings, name objects for them, and give them opportunities to explore their worlds.

—*Sandra Scarr*

DAY AND DATE: ....

	TIME	START (L or R)	MINUTES L	MINUTES R	AMOUNT EXPRESSED	SUPPLEMENT AMOUNT BREAST MILK	SUPPLEMENT AMOUNT FORMULA	OUTPUT WET	OUTPUT POOP
1									
2									
3									
4									
5									
6									
7									
8									
9									
10									
11									
12									
TOTALS:									

45 Days Old. If you'll be returning to the workplace or even working from home, you may soon be starting a search for a caregiver. At this point, it may be hard even to think about leaving your precious baby with someone else. You will feel better once you have found a caregiver you trust and with whom you have established a rapport.

Start by asking everyone you know for a referral. You might try a local nanny service, a website that matches families with nannies, or a county referral agency. Try to find someone who has experience with infants and respect for the breast-feeding relationship. When you find a good prospect, have a background check done, if you're not using an agency that provides this service. You might also arrange for the person to take a class in basic first-aid and infant CPR.

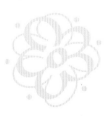

Making the decision to have a child is momentous. It is to decide forever to have your heart go walking around outside your body.

—*Elizabeth Stone*

_____

_____

_____

_____

_____

_____

_____

_____

_____

_____

_____

_____

_____

_____

_____

_____

_____

_____

_____

_____

	TIME	START (L or R)	MINUTES		AMOUNT EXPRESSED	SUPPLEMENT AMOUNT		OUTPUT	
			L	R		BREAST MILK	FORMULA	WET	POOP
1									
2									
3									
4									
5									
6									
7									
8									
9									
10									
11									
12									
TOTALS:									

DAY AND DATE: ....

46 Days Old. Once you are taking the baby out with you on errands and appointments, you need to feel comfortable nursing away from home. The prospect of nursing in public may seem daunting if you have only just mastered the skill of getting your baby positioned and latched on. But your baby's portability is one of the many perks of being a breastfeeding mom.

You'll expose less if you wear a blouse or sweater with a skirt or pants rather than a dress; pull the top up from the waist and use the baby to cover your skin. Some mothers practice in front of a mirror so they can see what others will see. If you want to be very discreet, search for tops designed for nursing, with slits for access to the breast, or a cape that is designed for covering up while breast-feeding.

While we try to teach our children all about life,
Our children teach us what life is all about.

—Angela Schwindt

DAY AND DATE: ....

	TIME	START (L or R)	MINUTES L	MINUTES R	AMOUNT EXPRESSED	SUPPLEMENT AMOUNT BREAST MILK	SUPPLEMENT AMOUNT FORMULA	OUTPUT WET	OUTPUT POOP
1									
2									
3									
4									
5									
6									
7									
8									
9									
10									
11									
12									
	TOTALS:								

47 Days Old. Are you already planning an extended road trip or air travel? Maybe the grandparents are urging you to visit, or maybe you have to take a business trip. Traveling with a baby, particularly if you're flying, takes some careful planning.

Forget scheduling the flight to coincide with nap time, since a delay or your baby's reactions to strange surroundings would likely defeat such a plan. Instead, arrange to travel at night or another time when the airports and flights are less busy. Pick a seat in the bulkhead, where you will have more room. Pack lightly but strategically. Arrange for a car seat at your destination or plan to bring your own, which may need to be checked as baggage. At many airports you can check a stroller at the gate, and it is ready for you when you step off the plane. Check with your airline for details.

Once you're on the plane, nurse during takeoff and descent to minimize the buildup of pressure in the baby's ears. At this age, most babies will doze off to the drone of the engines. *Bon voyage!*

Babies don't need a vacation but I still see them at the beach....
I'll go over to them and say, "What are you doing here, you've
never worked a day in your life!"

—*Steven Wright*

_____

_____

_____

_____

_____

_____

_____

_____

_____

_____

_____

_____

_____

_____

_____

_____

_____

_____

_____

_____

DAY AND DATE:

	TIME	START (L or R)	MINUTES L	MINUTES R	AMOUNT EXPRESSED	SUPPLEMENT AMOUNT BREAST MILK	SUPPLEMENT AMOUNT FORMULA	OUTPUT WET	OUTPUT POOP
1									
2									
3									
4									
5									
6									
7									
8									
9									
10									
11									
12									
	TOTALS:								

48 Days Old. You may notice that your breasts feel softer between feedings now (unless for some reason you miss a regular feeding), and that your milk doesn't let down as fast. If you are expressing your milk, you may find that you're producing a little less than you did in the early weeks. All of this is normal; you have adjusted to your baby's needs. It is still prudent, however, to nurse at least seven times a day. People may tell you otherwise, but your baby still needs to be fed at least once during the night to keep growing well and to keep up your milk supply.

We can see that the baby is as much an instrument of nourishment for us as we are for him.

—*Polly Berrien Berends*

DAY and DATE: ....

	TIME	START (L or R)	MINUTES L	MINUTES R	AMOUNT EXPRESSED	SUPPLEMENT AMOUNT BREAST MILK	SUPPLEMENT AMOUNT FORMULA	OUTPUT WET	OUTPUT POOP
1									
2									
3									
4									
5									
6									
7									
8									
9									
10									
11									
12									
TOTALS:									

49 Days Old. If you didn't start out with an abundant milk supply, if you have been supplementing your milk with formula, or if you have been frequently missing feedings, your milk production may be beginning to falter at this point. If you suspect this is happening, check your baby's weight. If the baby's weight gain has slowed, consider taking a "babymoon"—a day for both of you to rest in bed and nurse more often than usual.

Perhaps you have heard about herbs that increase milk production, including fenugreek, blessed thistle, shatavari, and fennel. These are available singly or mixed as teas, capsules, and tinctures. Check with a lactation specialist or doctor about their safety and about dosage. If you need a major boost to your milk supply, your doctor may even suggest a prescription medication.

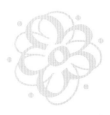

Breastfeeding is an unsentimental metaphor for how love works, in a way. You don't decide how much and how deeply to love—you respond to the beloved, and give with joy exactly as much as they want.

—*Marni Jackson*

DAY AND DATE: ....

	TIME	START (L or R)	MINUTES L	MINUTES R	AMOUNT EXPRESSED	SUPPLEMENT AMOUNT BREAST MILK	SUPPLEMENT AMOUNT FORMULA	OUTPUT WET	OUTPUT POOP
1									
2									
3									
4									
5									
6									
7									
8									
9									
10									
11									
12									
TOTALS:									

50 Days Old.

If you have decided to stay home with your baby rather than return to outside employment soon, you have the advantage of being available for most if not all of baby's feedings. But you may also feel isolated. Each day may seem made up of nothing but feedings, diaper changes, and erratic naptimes.

Try to take at least one outing a day, even if it is to the grocery store. Start a book club with other new mothers. Introduce yourself to other parents while you're out for walks, and then plan some neighborhood get-togethers. Take a mom-and-baby exercise class at the local community center, or join a monthly mothers-at-home group. Find ways to use your intellect and stay socially active while you reinvent yourself as a mother.

When you no longer bring home a paycheck, you may feed undervalued for your work as a mother. Talk these feelings over with your partner and friends. Your baby won't need your full-time care forever. Enjoy this interlude!

I looked on child rearing not only as a work of love and duty but as a profession that was fully as interesting and challenging as any honorable profession in the world and one that demanded the best I could bring to it.

—*Rose Kennedy*

DAY AND DATE:

	TIME	START (L or R)	MINUTES		AMOUNT EXPRESSED	SUPPLEMENT AMOUNT		OUTPUT	
			L	R		BREAST MILK	FORMULA	WET	POOP
1									
2									
3									
4									
5									
6									
7									
8									
9									
10									
11									
12									
TOTALS:									

51 Days Old. Some babies are so laid-back that they don't let you know when they're hungry. They may be content to spend a lot of time sucking on pacifiers. At night they may sleep for long intervals, and during the day they may go for three- to four-hour stretches without nursing. Sometimes the pattern starts when a mother puts her baby on a strict feeding schedule in an effort to foster regular, longer sleep intervals.

When feedings occur less frequently than seven times in twenty-four hours, slow weight gain and a low milk supply can result. If you find you are nursing less often than this, offer the breast more frequently during the day and evening. Instead of waiting until the baby is crying, look for signs of hunger such as finger sucking. Cut back on pacifier use, or eliminate it altogether. Consider having your baby's weight checked to be sure she is growing well.

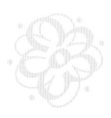

Loving a baby is a circular business, a kind of feedback loop.
The more you give the more you get and the more you get
the more you feel like giving.

—*Penelope Leach*

DAY AND DATE:

	TIME	START (L or R)	MINUTES		AMOUNT EXPRESSED	SUPPLEMENT AMOUNT		OUTPUT	
			L	R		BREAST MILK	FORMULA	WET	POOP
1									
2									
3									
4									
5									
6									
7									
8									
9									
10									
11									
12									
					TOTALS:				

52 Days Old. Do you find you are drifting away from the friends you had before you became a mother? Not only are you totally immersed in all things baby, but you may not have time for long phone chats and catch-up lunches. Childless friends may not understand this.

You may want to make an effort to revitalize these relationships. Call a friend you have had less contact with lately and plan a get-together. Arrange to meet at lunchtime for a quick brown-bag or take-out picnic, or invite her to drop by your house after work. If you'd like to host a little dinner party, have her bring the main dish or dessert. When you are together, avoid dominating the conversation with baby stories. Remember to ask what is new in your friend's life.

No one else on this planet is as interested in your baby
as you are.

—*Vicki Iovine*

_____

_____

_____

_____

_____

_____

_____

_____

_____

_____

_____

_____

_____

_____

_____

_____

_____

_____

_____

_____

DAY AND DATE:

	TIME	START (L or R)	MINUTES L	MINUTES R	AMOUNT EXPRESSED	SUPPLEMENT AMOUNT BREAST MILK	SUPPLEMENT AMOUNT FORMULA	OUTPUT WET	OUTPUT POOP
1									
2									
3									
4									
5									
6									
7									
8									
9									
10									
11									
12									
TOTALS:									

53 Days Old.

Nursing is probably a breeze for you now—but, then again, perhaps it isn't. If you are still struggling with some aspect of breastfeeding, be sure to seek assistance. A lactation specialist can help you identify the steps you might take to improve your situation.

If, despite your best efforts, you find that you are unable to feed your baby solely at the breast, this doesn't mean that you have to stop nursing entirely. You can continue to nurse while offering supplements as needed. Remember, any amount of breastfeeding is valuable for both you and your baby.

The world is full of women blindsided by the unceasing demands of motherhood, still flabbergasted by how a job can be terrific and torturous.

—*Anna Quindlen*

DAY AND DATE:

	TIME	START (L or R)	MINUTES L	R	AMOUNT EXPRESSED	SUPPLEMENT AMOUNT BREAST MILK	FORMULA	OUTPUT WET	POOP
1									
2									
3									
4									
5									
6									
7									
8									
9									
10									
11									
12									
TOTALS:									

54 Days Old. If your return to work is looming, it is time to prepare for those first days back. See if you can start with part-time hours, or at least return midweek so you'll have a break after the first few days.

Get a haircut if you need one, and pick out wardrobe pieces that will camouflage extra weight and make expressing easy. Figure out when and where you'll be expressing your milk. You might schedule an appointment with a lactation specialist for personal advice on making the transition back to work. Plan a dress rehearsal, or a few of them, with the baby's caregiver; leave the baby long enough to drop by the office or run other errands. While you're at the caregiver's, take some time to explain your baby's feeding routine.

It's normal to feel ambivalent about returning to a job. Naturally you are concerned about being away from your little one, but hopefully you're also excited to be returning to work that you love.

There is nothing to suggest that mothering cannot be shared
by several people.

—H. R. Schaffer

DAY AND DATE: ....

	TIME	START (L or R)	MINUTES L	MINUTES R	AMOUNT EXPRESSED	SUPPLEMENT AMOUNT BREAST MILK	SUPPLEMENT AMOUNT FORMULA	OUTPUT WET	OUTPUT POOP
1									
2									
3									
4									
5									
6									
7									
8									
9									
10									
11									
12									
TOTALS:									

55 Days Old. Without intending to, caregivers often overfeed babies. Trying to express enough to keep up with the overconsumption is the bane of working-and-nursing mothers.

A baby nearing two months needs 24 to 32 ounces every twenty-four hours, so a 3- to 4-ounce bottle should be an adequate replacement for each feeding you will miss. But babies tend to drink much more from bottles than they do at the breast. To prevent this, advise the caregiver to feed the baby slowly while holding her semi-upright, and to take frequent breaks during the feeding. Place some 2-ounce portions in the freezer in case your baby needs a snack or seems truly unsatisfied after a feeding.

To maintain your milk supply, express as often as possible when you are away, drink plenty of fluids, and nurse frequently when you and the baby are together.

A man's work is from sun to sun, but a mother's work
is never done.

—*Author Unknown*

DAY AND DATE: ....

	TIME	START (L or R)	MINUTES L	MINUTES R	AMOUNT EXPRESSED	SUPPLEMENT AMOUNT BREAST MILK	SUPPLEMENT AMOUNT FORMULA	OUTPUT WET	OUTPUT POOP
1									
2									
3									
4									
5									
6									
7									
8									
9									
10									
11									
12									
	TOTALS:								

56 Days Old. You are probably still struggling for more structure to your day and control over your time, especially if you are normally a very organized person. Life with a baby is a series of interruptions. It is easy to feel guilty about not being the best partner, best friend, best housekeeper and cook, and best daughter when you are spread so thin. Do your most pressing tasks early in the day, when your energy is highest. Carve out time for whatever makes you feel more accomplished—a morning walk or run, checking your email, or thoroughly cleaning the kitchen. In general, though, lower the bar. Make sure your partner is assisting in chores and errands; remember that you're a mother, not a maid.

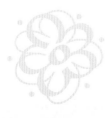

A woman without a child may have a house that shines,
but a woman with a child has a face that shines.

—*Indian proverb*

DAY AND DATE: ....

	TIME	START (L or R)	MINUTES L	MINUTES R	AMOUNT EXPRESSED	SUPPLEMENT AMOUNT BREAST MILK	SUPPLEMENT AMOUNT FORMULA	OUTPUT WET	OUTPUT POOP
1									
2									
3									
4									
5									
6									
7									
8									
9									
10									
11									
12									
TOTALS:									

57 Days Old. Parenting involves a lot of choices and experimentation. Some of us end up raising our children much as we were raised, and others do the opposite. People may tell you that your baby should be on a strict schedule for feeding and sleeping by now, and that she should learn to put herself to sleep by "crying it out." Most child-development experts, however, disagree. Babies cry to express real needs, and when their needs are met they are not "spoiled." Do what feels right to you and your partner, and trust your instincts. You are the experts on your baby.

Parents have become so convinced that educators know what is best for their children that they forget that they themselves are really the experts.

—*Marian Wright Edelman*

DAY AND DATE:

	TIME	START (L or R)	MINUTES L	R	AMOUNT EXPRESSED	SUPPLEMENT AMOUNT BREAST MILK	FORMULA	OUTPUT WET	POOP
1									
2									
3									
4									
5									
6									
7									
8									
9									
10									
11									
12									
TOTALS:									

58 Days Old. The two-month visit to your baby's doctor is coming up. This visit will probably be longer than the preceding one, since the first vaccines will be given. Think about what questions you might ask, write them down in this diary, and bring it along. The doctor can be a good source of information about many things, including local mothers' groups and lactation specialists. If possible, bring along your partner or a friend to take notes, to hold the baby, or to help you later recall medical explanations.

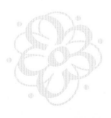

The child must know that he is a miracle, that since the beginning of the world there hasn't been, and until the end of the world there will not be, another child like him.

—*Pablo Casals*

DAY AND DATE: ....

	TIME	START (L or R)	MINUTES L	R	AMOUNT EXPRESSED	SUPPLEMENT AMOUNT BREAST MILK	FORMULA	OUTPUT WET	POOP
1									
2									
3									
4									
5									
6									
7									
8									
9									
10									
11									
12									
TOTALS:									

59 Days Old.

Fatigue is universal among new mothers. By the end of the second month post partum, you may be feeling better rested, but it will be a long time before you feel you've caught up on missed sleep. If you are still dragging most of the time, though, you should examine your diet and the amount of exercise you are getting. Good food and vigorous activity will not replace sleep, but they will help you function better. If you are truly exhausted, have your doctor check your iron and thyroid levels. If you are feeling despair and worthlessness, seek evaluation for postpartum depression.

You may be encouraged by the "12-pound rule," which says that babies begin sleeping "through the night" when they reach 12 pounds. This is an oft-repeated but inaccurate promise, so don't get your hopes up. Many babies, however, begin to stretch out intervals between night feedings at about two months of age.

A baby will make love stronger, days shorter, nights longer, bankroll smaller, home happier, clothes shabbier, the past forgotten, and the future worth living for.

—*Anonymous*

DAY AND DATE: ....

| | TIME | START (L or R) | MINUTES | | AMOUNT EXPRESSED | SUPPLEMENT AMOUNT | | OUTPUT | |
			L	R		BREAST MILK	FORMULA	WET	POOP
1									
2									
3									
4									
5									
6									
7									
8									
9									
10									
11									
12									
TOTALS:									

60 Days Old. As you come to the end of this diary, you may be surprised at how fast these first two months have flown by. You have changed hundreds of diapers and nursed your baby as many times. You have survived sleepless nights and fuzzy days. You have surmounted the fears and frustrations of very early parenthood, and you and your partner have created a family. Congratulate each other for this and for all the milestones you have met.

In nurturing another being with your body before and after birth, you have joined a sorority of women who have learned what it means to love someone more than they love themselves. Your life will never be just your own again, but it has been enriched beyond measure.

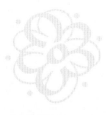

It will be gone before you know it. The fingerprints on the wall
appear higher and higher. Then suddenly they disappear.

—*Dorothy Evslin*

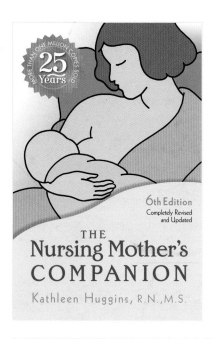

**The Nursing Mother's Companion
25th Anniversary Edition**
By Kathleen Huggins
  The sixth edition of this classic,
  comprehensive guide to breastfeeding
  has been extensively revised and
  updated. It includes easy-reference
  "survival guides" and an invaluable
  appendix on the safety of various
  drugs during breastfeeding.

More books by Kathleen Huggins from The Harvard Common Press:

The Nursing Mother's Guide to Weaning
By Kathleen Huggins and Linda Ziedrich
  This book explores the emotional, hygienic, and nutritional concerns of
  weaning a child at any age, from early infancy through the fourth year
  and beyond. Included is advice on introducing bottles and solid foods
  and on solving breastfeeding difficulties that often bring nursing to a
  premature close.

Nursing Mother, Working Mother
By Kathleen Huggins and Gale Pryor
  This award-winning guide expertly addresses all the issues facing
  working mothers who want to continue breastfeeding, such as pumping
  and storing milk, keeping up the milk supply, and the legal rights of
  employees with regard to breastfeeding.

25 Things Every Nursing Mother Needs to Know
By Kathleen Huggins and Jan Ellen Brown
  This encouraging, sometimes humorous book provides 25 essential tips
  for getting breastfeeding off to a good start.

See www.nursingmotherscompanion.com for more information.